Essential Oils for Weight Loss

Ultimate Beginners Guide to Losing Weight, Burning Fat, and Getting Healthy

Farrah Dale

Table of Contents

Introduction

Many of us struggle with our weight. We all know that eating right and excercising are the main ways to healthy weight loss. But what if I told you there was a secret weapon? An all natural way to boost your metabolism, curb cravings, and even reduce cellulite. This secret weapon comes straight from mother nature in the form of essential oils. Essential oils are natural, have no side effects, and have been used for centuries. Oh, and did I mention they smell good too.

This book is written with the beginner in mind. Inside you will learn what essential oils are and where they come from. You will also learn how to use them and which ones work the best to help you lose weight. You won't only learn what oils to use, but WHY and HOW they work on the body! Essential oils work together on your mind, body, and spirit to create real and complete results unlike other methods.

I would also like to mention that this book is not trying to sell you anything, tell you what brands to buy, or advertise a specific product. There are no ulterior motives here. It is written to give real advice on how to aid your weight loss as well as how essential oils can also improve your health and even your skin. You can get started with just one bottle of essential oil. There are also a ton of recipes inside you can use to create things like anti-cellulite rubs, weight loss bath blends and much more.

I hope you enjoy this book and can't wait to hear about your results!

Chapter 1

What are Essential Oils?

Ancient manuscripts have dated the use essential oils all around the world as far back as 4500 BC. For thousands of years, essential oils have been used for medicinal and religious purposes, as well as for cooking, aromatherapy and perfumery. In modern times, various studies and research show that essential oils provide therapeutic and health benefits to humans and animals. But unlike modern drugs, using essential oils have little or no side-effects at all.

The term "essential oil" is derived from the original term "quintessential oil" that refers to the highly concentrated, complex, powerful, natural, and fragrant substances that are extracted from plants. These distinct substances are vital for plants to evolve, grow, and adapt to their surroundings. They also help defend plants from disease, insects, and harsh environmental conditions. Also referred to as the essence of the plant, essential oils not only protect, but also give the plant its aroma.

How Are These Oils Extracted?

Essential oils are derived through various processes using plant parts - roots, leaves, bark, flowers, fruits, seeds, and other natural resources.

Distillation

The most common essential oil extraction process is steam distillation. Raw plant material, consisting of plant leaves, flowers, and more, is placed into an alembic or distillation apparatus over water. The water is heated. As the steam from the hot water goes up, it passes through the raw plant materials, vaporizing the volatile compounds of the plant. The compound vapors will flow through a coil, where they will cool and condense back into liquid. Finally, it drips and collects in the receiving vessel at the end of the coil. Once in the collector, the essential oil will separate from the water (aqueous portion or the hydrosol).

Cold Press or Expression

This method of extraction is used particularly for citrus fruits. Cold press is used for citrus fruits because the large quantities of oil from these fruits are found in their peel. When you peel a lemon or an orange, you can actually squeeze the oil from the peel. In the old days, the rinds of citrus fruits are hand squeezed into sponges to collect the oil. Nowadays, with the help of centrifugal technology, it is easier to extract essential oil without the need to hand press the skin of the fruit.

Enfleurage

This method of extraction mostly used for flowers and is the oldest method. However, it is seldom used today.

Cold Enfleurage

Animal fat (usually tallow or lard) is smeared in a chassis or a framed plate of glass. Flower petals, usually rose petals, are placed on top of the fat and is allowed to set for about 1-3 days. During this time, the scent of the flowers will diffuse into the fat. The flowers are replaced with fresh petals until the fat has reached the desired concentration of fragrance.

Hot Enfleurage

Solid fats are heated. Botanical material is then stirred into the heated fat. Spent materials are strained repeatedly and replaced with fresh material until the fat is saturated with the desired concentration of fragrance.

Solvent Extraction or Absolute Method

As its name suggests, this is how absolutes are made - highly concentrated essential oils with true, unadulterated aroma that are used in perfumery. The raw aromatic plant material is macerated and covered with a volatile solvent, like hexane, which softens the plant material and extracts the essential oil into an aromatic paste. After the volatile substance is evaporated, the paste or also called concrete substance, is further diluted into ethyl alcohol, which undergoes filtration process to further eliminate the waxy residues. The filtered solution undergoes a steam distillation that separates the aromatic essential oils from the alcoholic solution.

CO2 Extraction

This process of extraction is another method to extract absolute oils. Carbon dioxide or CO2 (gas under pressure) is used as the solvent. This method of extraction is expensive and is mainly used to extract essential oils used for drink, food, herbal industries, and body care.

Infused Oil (Homemade)

Although this will not extract pure or absolute essential oil, this method is an easy and affordable way to create your own herbal-based oil for massage. Pour carrier oil into a jar, about 1/2 full. Add in plant materials of your choice (herbs, orange peel, rose, jasmine, lemon peel) until the jar is full. Allow the plant material to soak in the carrier oil for 2 weeks in a dark, cold place, allowing the plant to release its properties into the oil.

Here are a few tips if you want to make your own infused oil.

- Sterilize the jar. Make sure it is completely dry, without a single drop of water inside because water encourages the growth of mold and bacteria.

- When using fresh herbs, make sure you wash them to get rid of bugs and dirt. Allow them to completely dry, meaning there is no trace of water on the plant, but do not allow the plants to become dried herbs. Chop the herbs to help release the essential oils.

- After two weeks, strain your infused oil using cheesecloth. Pour into clean bottles and store in cool, dark place or in the refrigerator.

- Infused oils will last for about 6 months.

- You can also add to your infused oil with vitamin E. Just break or prick several capsules with a needle and pour contents into your infused oil.

Chapter 2

The Benefits of Essential Oils

Like most plant-derived remedies, the full therapeutic potential of essential oils is yet to be fully understood. Although numerous medicinal herbs and essential oils have been utilized since ancient times, there is still a great deal to be discovered. Essential oils cover a wide field of activities and can stimulate the various systems of the body while relaxing and sedating others. To gain clearer understanding of the therapeutic properties of essential oils, it is important to take an overall view of the of the body's systems and how essential oils can help benefit that particular system of the body.

The Skin

Skin problems are often the body's way of saying that there is a deeper problem, such as hormonal imbalance, emotional or nervous difficulties, or build-up of toxins in the blood.

Since essential oils can impart their scent in water, absorbed through the skin via osmosis, and soluble in alcohol and other oils, they are ideal ingredients for general skin care, cosmetics, and treatment for specific skin diseases.

Actions					
Antiseptic	Anti-inflammatory	Fungicidal	Granulation Stimulating or Cicatrising (healing) Agents	Deodorants	Insect Repellents and Parasiticides
Cuts	Eczema	Athlete's	Burns	Excessive	Lice
Insect bites	Infected	foot	Cuts	perspiration	Fleas
Spots	wounds	Candida	Scars	Cleaning	Scabies
	Bumps	Ringworm	Stretch	Wounds	Ticks
	Bruises		marks		Mosquitos
					Ants
					Moths
Essential Oil					
Thyme	Roman and	Lavender	Lavender	Bergamot	Spike
Sage	German	Tea tree	Chamomile	Lavender	Lavender
Eucalyptus	chamomile	Myrrh	Rose	Thyme	Garlic
Tea tree	Lavender	Patchouli	Neroli	Juniper	Geranium
clove	Yarrow	Sweet	Frankincense	Cypress	Citronella
Lavender		marjoram	Geranium	Spanish sage	Eucalyptus
Lemon				Lemongrass	Clove
					Camphor
					Atlas cedarwood

The Circulation, Joints, and Muscles

Essential oils are readily absorbed into the bloodstream through the skin and the mucosa, affecting the body's circulation as a whole. Oils with warming effect or rubefacient effects are better when applied in the local area of blood circulation that, in turn, affects the inner organs as well. These oils are often used to relieve inflammation, expanding the blood vessels and moving blood quickly, reducing swelling.

One essential oil in particular, the hyssop, has a regulating or balancing effect, stimulating the blood if it is sluggish and reducing the blood pressure if it is too high.

Actions					
Hypotensives	Hypertensives	Rubefacients	Depurative or Antitoxic Agents	Lymphatic Stimulants	Circulatory Tonics and Astringents
High blood pressure Palpitations Stress	Poor circulation Chilblains Listlessness	Rheumatism of the joints Muscular stiffness Sciatica Lumbago	Arthritis Gout Congestion Skin eruptions	Cellulitis Obesity Water retention	Swellings Inflammations Varicose veins
Essential Oil					
Sweet marjoram, Ylang-Ylang Lavender Lemon	Rosemary Spike lavender Eucalyptus Peppermint Thyme	Black pepper Juniper Rosemary Camphor Sweet marjoram	Juniper Lemon Fennel Lovage	Grapefruit Lime Fennel Lemon Mandarin White birch	Cypress Yarrow Lemon

The Respiratory System

Lung, throat, and nose conditions respond well to essential oil treatment. Inhalation is the best method since the therapeutic effects will be exhaled directly into the lungs. Inhalation also allows the essential oil to be absorbed into the blood faster.

Actions			
Expectorants	Antispasmodics	Balsamic agents	Antiseptics
Catarrh	Colic	Colds	Flu
Sinusitis	Asthma	Chills Congestion	Colds
Coughs	Dry cough		Sore throat
Bronchitis	Whooping Cough		Tonsillitis
			Gingivitis
Essential Oil			
Eucalyptus	Hyssop	Benzoin	Thyme
Pine	Cypress	Frankincense	Sage
Thyme	Atlas cedarwood	Tolu balsam	Eucalyptus
Myrrh	Bergamot	Peru balsam	Hyssop
Sandalwood	Chamomile	Myrrhs	Pine
Fennel	Cajeput		Cajeput
			Tea tree
			Borneol

The Digestive System

Although it is strictly not recommended to take essential oils orally, external applications can benefit the digestive system. However, the external application of essential oil is limited. Make sure you are using the highest quality oils if you will be taking them orally.

Actions				
Antispasmodics	Carminatives and Stomachics	Cholagogues	Hepatics	Aperitifs
Spasm	Flatulent	Increasing the flow of bile	Liver congestion	Loss of appetite
Pain	dyspepsia			
Indigestion	Aerophagia			Anorexia
	Nausea	Stimulating the gall bladder	Jaundice	
Essential Oil				
Chamomile	Angelica	Caraway	Lemon	Aniseed
Caraway	Basil	Lavender	Lime	Angelica
Fennel	Fennel	Peppermint	Rosemary	Orange
Orang	Chamomile	Borneol	Peppermint	Ginger
Peppermint	Peppermint			Garlic
Lemon balm	Mandarin			
Aniseed				
Cinnamon				

The Endocrine and Genito-urinary Systems

Similar to the digestive system, the reproductive organs can benefit from essential oil via absorption through the skin and into the bloodstream.

Actions					
Antispasmodics	Emmenagogues	Uterine Tonics and Regulators	Antiseptic and Bactericidal Agents	Galactagogues	Aphrodisiacs
Menstrual cramp (dysmenorrhea) Labor pains	Scanty periods Lack of periods or amenorrhea	Pregnancy Excess menstruation or menorrhagia PMT	Leucorrhoea Vaginal pruritis Thrush	Increasing milk flow	Impotence Frigidity
Essential Oil					
Sweet marjoram Chamomile Clary sage Jasmine Lavender	Chamomile Fennel Hyssop Juniper Sweet marjoram Peppermint	Clary sage Jasmine Rose Myrrh Frankincense Lemon balm	Bergamot Chamomile Myrrh Rose Tea tree	Fennel Jasmine Anise Lemongrass	Black pepper Cardomon Clary sage Neroli Jasmine Rose Sandalwood Patchouli Ylang-Ylang

ACTIONS		
Anaphrodisiacs	**Adrenal Stimulants**	**Urinary Antiseptics**
Reducing sexual desire	Anxiety Stress-related conditions	Cystitis Urethritis
Essential Oil		
Sweet marjoram Camphor	Basil, Rosemary, Borneol, Geranium, Pine, Sage, avory	Chamomile, Sandalwood, Bergamot, Tea tree

The Immune System

Fundamentally, all essential oils have bacterial properties, stimulating the production of white blood cells, preventing and treating infectious illness.

ACTIONS		
Bactericidal and Antiviral Agents (prophylactics)	**Febrifuge Agents**	**Sudorifics and Diaphoretics**
Colds Flu	Reducing fever and temperature	Promoting sweating Eliminating toxins
Essential Oil		
Tea Tree, Niaouli, Cajeput, Basil, Eucalyptus, Lavender, Bergamot, Clove, Camphor, Rosemary	Basil, Angelica, Thyme, Peppermint, Lemon, Sage, Tea Tree, Eucalyptus	Thyme, Rosemary, Chamomile, Hyssop,

The Nervous System

According to research, depending on their properties, some essential oils have sedative effects (such as lemon, bergamot, chamomile, lavender, sandalwood, and sweet marjoram) while others have stimulating effects (such as neroli, peppermint, jasmine, clove, basil, and ylang-ylang).

Scents that have "uplifting" or "relaxing" aromas often have more to do with the emotional response and scent description instead of the physiological effect. For example, lemon and lemon balm have a sedating effect on the nervous system, but uplifting to the senses. On the other hand, ylang-ylang, jasmine, and neroli have stimulating effects yet relaxing and soothing to the senses.

ACTIONS		
Sedatives	**Stimulants**	**Nerve tonics (nervines)**
Nervous tension, Insomnia, Stress,	Convalescence, nervous fatigue, lack of strength	Strengthening the nervous system as a whole
Essential Oil		
Bergamot, Chamomile, Lavender, Sandalwood, Lemon Sweet Marjoram, Hops, Balm, Valerian, Lemon	Basil, Peppermint, Jasmine, Neroli, Ylang Ylang, Rosemary, Angelica	Clary Sage, Chamomile, Lavender, Juniper, Rosemary Marjoram,

The Mind

This area in the least understood concerning the benefits of essential oil. There is no doubt that essential oils have been used throughout history for their power to influence the state of the emotions and the mind.

According to various research, when we inhale essential oil fragrance, the scent molecules travel up to the nose, where they are registered and stimulate the limbic system or the part of the brain that is directly connected to the parts of the brain that control blood pressure, heart rate, memory, breathing, hormone balance, and stress levels. Furthermore, the scent of essential oils stimulates the brain to produce neurochemicals and the hormones that affect the body, producing effects.

Chapter 3

Best 6 Essential Oils for Weight Loss

Among the numerous essential oils available, these six are at the top oils for weight loss. Let's get to know them better, shall we?

Grapefruit Essential Oil

The oil in this sour to sweet tasting citrus fruit has a fresh, bitter, sweet, and citrus aroma. Like most citrus fruits, grapefruit is high in vitamin C and helps protect against illnesses and infections.

Extraction	Actions	Principal Constituents	Safety Data	Blends Well With
Cold fresh from the fresh peel	Tonic Stimulant (lymphatic and digestive) Diuretic Depurative Bactericidal Astringent Antitoxic Antiseptic	Cadinene Citronellal Esters (coumarins and furocoumarins) Geraniol Limonene (90 %) Neral Paradisiol Sinensal	Has a short life, oxidizes quickly Non-irritant Non-phototoxic Non-sensitizing Non-toxic	Bergamot Cardomon Cypress Geranium Lavender Lemon Neroli Palmarosa Rosemary Other spice oils

Home/ Aromatherapy Use			
Skin Care	Muscles, Joints, and Circulation	Immune System	Nervous System
Acne	Exercise	Colds	Depression
Oily and congested skin	preparation	Chills	Headaches
Tones tissues and skin	Cellulitis	Flu	Nervous Exhaustion
Stimulates hair growth	Obesity		Performance
	Muscle fatigue		Stress
	Water retention		
	Stiffness		

How It Aids Weight Loss

Naringenin

According to the research conducted by the Massachusetts General Hospital and the University of Jerusalem, grapefruit contains naringenin, an antioxidant that can possibly treat type 2 diabetes and cholesterol. Naringenin helps the liver break down fat and increases the body's insulin sensitivity, similar to the effects of antidiabetic and lipid-lowering drugs. This antioxidant also protects liver from damage.

Nootkatone

This natural chemical compound stimulates a specific enzyme (AMPK to be exact), which controls the body's metabolic rate and energy levels, reducing weight gain, decreasing body fat, and improving physical performance.

Soluble Fiber

Rich in pectin, a soluble fiber, it helps lower the body's cholesterol levels.

Antioxidant

Aside from naringenin, grapefruit contains lycopene, a phytochemical that has powerful antioxidant properties that fights free radical that damages the cells of the body.

Lemon Essential Oil

This pale green to yellow fruit has a clean, light, slightly sour, sugary citrus scent. The peel and the juice of lemon is widely used as a seasoning. It is high in vitamin C, B, and A, and is known as an all-cure, particularly to infectious illness.

Extraction	Actions	Principal Constituents	Safety Data	Blends Well With
Cold press from the outer part of the fresh peel	Vermifuge Tonic Stimulates white corpuscles Rubefacient Insecticidal Hypotensive Haemostatic Febrifuge Diuretic Diaphoretic Depurative Cicatrisant Carminative Bactericidal Astringent Antitoxic Antispasmodic Antiseptic Antiscorbutic Antirheumatic antisclerotic Antimicrobial Anti-anaemic	Bergamotene Citral Citronellal Geraniol Limonene (approx. 70 %) Linalol Myrcene Nonanol Octanol Pinenes Sabinene Terpinene	Non-toxic Can cause sensitization reactions or dermal irritation in some individuals apply moderately Phototoxic – do not apply on skin and exposed to direct sunlight	Benzoin, Chamomile Elemi Eucalyptus Fennel Geranium Juniper Labdanum Lavandin Lavender Neroli Oakmoss Olibanum Rose Sandalwood Ylang-Ylang Other citrus oils

Home/ Aromatherapy Use				
Skin Care	Muscles, Joints, and Circulation	Respiratory System	Digestive System	Immune System
Acne	Arthritis	Asthma	Dyspepsia	Colds
Anemia	Cellulitis	Throat		Flu
Brittle nails	High blood	infections		Fever
Boils	pressure	bronchitis		Infections
Chilblains	Nosebleeds	Catarrh		
Corns	Obesity			
Cuts	(congestion)			
Greasy skin	Poor			
Herpes	circulation			
Insect bites	Rheumatism			
Mouth ulcers				
Spots				
Varicose veins				
warts				

How It Aids Weight Loss

D-Limonene

Lemon essential oil contains 70 percent limonene. Also called terpene, this nutrient oil is a natural compound with potent anti-inflammatory and antioxidant properties. Limonene improves digestion, cleanses fat, reduces appetite, increases metabolism, and helps clear cholesterol. Limonene also works by increasing lipolysis or the breakdown of fats in the body.

Raises Norepinephrine Levels

The scent of lemon increases levels of the neurotransmitter and stress hormone called Norepinephrine. This, in turn, increases blood flow to the brain, improving brain function, increasing the blood flow and heart rate of the body, and allowing the muscles to work better and faster.

Peppermint Essential Oil

This essential oil extracted from the leaves of hybrid mint, a cross between watermint and spearmint has a powerful, fresh, hot, very minty, herbaceous, sweet scent.

Extraction	Actions	Principal Constituents	Safety Data	Blends Well With
Steam distilled from the flowering plant	Tonic Cytophylactic Anti-infective Antiseptic Decongestant Antibiotic Antifungal Antidepressant Anti-toxic Aphrodisiac Astringent Calmative Nervine Anti-inflammatory to the prostate and the nerves	Menthol (70%) Menthone Menthyl acetate Neomenthol 1,8-Cineole Menthofuran	Avoid while pregnant and in epilepsy Can cause skin irritation Avoid with homeopathics	Basil Benzoin Black pepper Cypress Eucalyptus Geranium Grapefruit Juniper Lavender Lemon Marjoram Niaouli Pine Ravensara Rosemary Tea tree

How It Aids Weight Loss

Containing up to 70% menthol, peppermint essential oil has the following benefits:

Suppresses Appetite

A study conducted in 2008 revealed that inhaling the strong scent of peppermint essential oil lowers hunger levels and helps the individual decrease food consumption.

Improves and Helps Digestion

This oil helps calm down the body's gastrointestinal tract, allowing healthier bowel movement. To put it simply, it helps keeps things flowing and moving, alleviating constipation, reducing bloating, and improving bile flow. In turn, allowing food to be digested in the body faster.

Relaxes the Body

When the body is stressed, there is an increase in the cortisol level, slowing down metabolism. Inhaling the aroma of peppermint essential oil decreases the fatigue and stress levels, soothing, calming, reducing stress, and thus, keeping the body's metabolism on track.

Cinnamon Essential Oil (Leaf)

This oil has a sweet, warm, flat, earthy spice, dry, tenacious scent.

Extraction	Actions	Principal Constituents	Safety Data	Blends Well With
Steam distilled from leaves	Vermifuge Stomachic Stimulant (cardiac, circulatory, respiratory) Spasmolytic Refrigerant Parasiticide Orexigenic Haemostatic Emmenagogue Digestive Carminative Astringent Aphrodisiac Antispasmodic Antiseptic Antiputrescent Antimicrobial Antidote (to poison) Antidiarrhoeal Anthelmintic	Eugenol (80–96%) Eugenol acetate Cinnamaldehyde (3%) Benzyl benzoate Linalool Safrol	Relatively non-toxic Possibly irritant due to cinnamaldehyde Eugenol, it's major component, can cause irritation to the mucous membranes: use moderately	Olibanum, Benzoin, Bergamot Cardamom Clove Frankincense Ginger Grapefruit Lemon Mandarin Mandarin Marjoram Nutmeg Orange Peppermint Peru balsam Oriental-type mixtures Petitgrain Rose Vanilla Ylang-Ylang

Home/ Aromatherapy Use					
Skin Care	Muscles, Joints, and Circulation	Genito-Urinary System	Digestive System	Immune System	Nervous System
Lice Scabies Tooth and gum care Warts Wasp stings	Rheumatism Poor circulation	Frigidity Child birth (stimulates contractions) Leucorrhoea Metrorrhagia Scanty periods	Anorexia Colitis Diarrhoea Dyspepsia Intestinal infection Sluggish digestion Spasm	Colds Chills Flu Infectious disease	Stress related conditions Nervous exhaustion Debility

How It Aids Weight Loss

Eugenol

Containing 80-96% eugenol, this essential oil an antibacterial and it helps promote good digestion, alleviating upset stomach, nausea, and diarrhea.

Increases Metabolic Activity

Cinnamon helps remove blood impurities and improves blood circulation. This response helps supply adequate oxygen to the cells of the body and increases the body's metabolic rate.

Heightens Insulin Sensitivity

Cinnamon extract increases the rate of blood glucose uptake in the body, facilitating conversion of fat into energy.

Bergamot Essential Oil

This essential oil has a fresh, lively, spicy, floral, fruity, sweet, citrus aroma.

Extraction	Actions	Principal Constituents	Safety Data	Blends Well With
Cold press from the inside peel of a nearly ripe fruit	Vulnerary Vermifuge Tonic Stomachic Stimulant Rubefacient Parasiticide Laxative Febrifuge Diuretic Digestive Deodorant Carminative Antitoxic Antispasmodic Antiseptic (pulmonary, genito-urinary) Antidepressant Anthelmintic Analgesic	300 compounds, including mainly: Linalyl acetate (30–60%), Linalool (11–22 %) Other alcohols, terpenes, sesquiterpenes, alkanes and furocoumarins (including bergapten, 0.30–0.39%)	Certain furocoumarins, particularly bergapten, have phototoxic effects on human skin – avoid exposure to sunlight when using. Using bergapten-free versions are relatively non-irritant and non-toxic.	lavender, neroli, jasmine, cypress, geranium, lemon, chamomile, juniper, coriander violet Chamomile, citrus oils, coriander, cypress, geranium, helichrysum, jasmine, juniper, lavender, lemon balm, neroli, nutmeg, rose, sandalwood, vetiver, violet ylang-ylang

Home/ Aromatherapy Use					
Skin Care	Respiratory System	Genito-Urinary System	Digestive System	Immune System	Nervous System
Acne	Halitosis	Cystitis	Loss of	Fever	Depression
Boils	Mouth	Leucorrhoea	appetite	Flu	Anxiety
Cold sores	infections	Pruritis	Flatulence	Colds	Stress-
Eczema	Sore throat	Thrush		Infectious	related
Insect	Tonsillitis			diseases	conditions
repellent					
Insect bites					
Oily					
complexion					
Psoriasis					
Scabies					
Spots					
Varicose					
Ulcers					
Wounds					

How It Aids Weight Loss

Helps Combat Overeating

Like peppermint, bergamot stimulates the endocrine system, producing calming and relaxing feelings. Bergamot essential oil helps alleviate emotional stress, reducing the common symptom of "comfort eating" or overeating.

Stimulates Hormone Secretion

Bergamot increases the bile, digestive juices, and insulin, helping maintain and boost the body's metabolic rate.

Regulates Cholesterol and Blood Sugar

Bergamot reduces the enzyme (HMG-CoA), an enzyme connected to cholesterol production of the liver, lowering the levels of bad cholesterol in the blood and raising good cholesterol. The reduced amount of HMG-CoA also lowers the levels of blood sugar in the body.

Fennel Essential Oil (Sweet Fennel)

Sweet Fennel essential oil has an almost peppery, sweet, earthy aroma.

Extraction	Actions	Principal Constituents	Safety Data	Blends Well With
Steam distilled from the seeds	Vermifuge Tonic Stomachic Stimulant (circulatory) Splenic Orexigenic Laxative Galactagogue Expectorant Emmenagogue Diuretic Depurative Carminative Aperitif Antispasmodic Antiseptic Antimicrobial Anti-inflammatory	Anethole (50–60%) Limonene Phellandrene Pinene Anisic acid Anisic aldehyde Camphene Limonene	Non-irritant Relatively non-toxic Narcotic in large doses Not to be sued during pregnancy or by epileptics Use moderately	Bergamot Black pepper Cardamom Cypress Dill Fir Geranium Ginger Grapefruit Juniper Lavender Lemon Mandarin Marjoram Niaouli Orange Pine Ravensara Rose Rosemary Sandalwood Tangerine Ylang-Ylang

Home/ Aromatherapy Use				
Skin Care	Muscles, Joints, and Circulation	Genito-Urinary System	Digestive System	Respiratory System
Bruises Dull Oily, mature complexions Pyorrhoea	Cellulitis Obesity Edema Rheumatism	Amenorrhea Insufficient milk (in nursing mothers) Menopausal problems	Anorexia Colic Constipation Dyspepsia Flatulence Hiccough Nausea	Asthma Bronchitis

How It Aids Weight Loss

Melatonin

This hormone regulates the body's natural circadian rhythm for a more restful sleep. Melatonin increases the amount of "beige fat" in the body, which burns off energy, rather than build up "white fat" that is stored in the body.

Reduces Hunger Pangs

Fennel has an anti-spasmodic effect that helps relieve hunger pangs.

Diuretic

Fennel increases the frequency of urination, reducing the water weight of the body, eliminating stagnant fluids, toxins, and fats. When massaged on the body, it boosts the circulation of the blood and draws the excess water away from the tissues, minimizing cellulite.

Carminative Nature

To put it simply, it helps relieve and prevent flatulence. It also smooths the stomach and intestine muscles, preventing indigestion, belching, nausea, and abdominal bloating. As we know too well by now, good digestion helps weight loss.

Chapter 4

How to Use Essential Oils

There are four ways to use essential oil to aid weight loss and each method will be described below. I know. You are excited to try everything that you've learned so far. Hold your horses! Before you go jumping ahead, please make sure you read Chapter 6: Essential Oil Safety and precautions. When used incorrectly, you may untowardly put yourself at risk rather than reap the benefits of using essential oils.

Inhalation

Inhalation of essential oils triggers various desired responses and heightens the senses. In this case, we are using Essential oils to initiate various weight loss reactions in the body. Below are several inhalation techniques you can choose from.

Direct Inhalation

To put it simply, just open your bottle of essential oil and breathe in a whiff. Or you can do any of the following instead:

• Put a few drops of oil on a cotton ball. Place it in front of a fan or a vent.

• Place a cotton ball with a few drops of oil in a small zip-lock bag. You can carry this around with you.

- Pour a few drops of oil in your handkerchief or a tissue.

- Pour a few drops of oil on your pillow at night.

Inhalers

If you have a used or empty inhaler tube, you can place a cotton ball inside and pour a few drops of oil into the cotton. This is a pretty easy way to carry the aroma with you all the time and prevent the scent from spreading when you are using it in public. Refresh the inhaler by adding a drop of two when needed.

Room Sprays

Not only will this help you lose weight, this method also removes unwanted odors and disinfects your home.

1. Pour warm water into a plant mister.

2. Pour a few drops of essential oil. Shake, shake, shake.

3. Spray in your bedroom before you sleep at night or anywhere in the house where you usually spend time.

Just be sure to avoid spraying over fabrics, furniture, or any surface that could be damaged by water.

Steam Inhalation

1. Add about 5 drops of your preferred essential oil into a bowl filled with hot water.

2.   Using a large towel, like a tent, cover your head and the bowl.

3.   Breathe in deeply and slowly for 60 seconds – then repeat.

If you notice any irritation, stop immediately.

Some saunas actually offer a steaming hot bath where you can inhale a certain amount of essential oil. This is one way of inhaling essential oil. However, the concentration will not be as concentrated. On the other hand, essential oil inhalation in saunas helps clear the complexion and unclog the pores.

Humidifier Inhalation

1.   Fill a humidifier with water.

2.   Sprinkle a few drops of your preferred essential oil a small cloth or a tissue.

3.   Place the cloth or the tissue in front of the escaping humidifier steam. Enjoy the scent.

Please do not directly drop oil in the humidifier. The oil will not rise with the water, floating on top of it instead. This can damage the humidifier.

Diluted With Carrier Oil

Carrier, or also called base oils, are often used with essential oil. Why? Basically, pure essential oil is too concentrated and cannot be applied undiluted to the skin. Mixing with base oils is a great way to dilute the essential oil for safe application on the skin. This method also allows the essential oil to be spread over a larger area and be absorbed evenly through the skin. Likewise, essential oils are quite expensive. Diluting allows you to use smaller amounts. Nevertheless, one or two drops are often more beneficial than larger amounts and is certainly safer and less likely to cause adverse reactions.

Carrier (Base) Oils

The most popular base oils include the following. Choose from any for your dilutions.

Base Oil	Skin Type	Relieves	Base Oil Use
Sweet Almond	All skin types	Soreness, dryness, inflammation, itching	100 percent
Apricot Kernel	All skin types, particularly sensitive, aging, dry, and inflamed skin		100 percent
Avocado	All skin types, particularly dehydrated and dry skin	Eczema	Additive to a base, not exceeding 10 percent
Borage	All skin types	Menopausal problems, psoriasis, multiple sclerosis, eczema, heart disease, and prematurely aged skin; regenerate and stimulate skin	Additive to a base, not exceeding 10 percent
Coconut	All skin types, especially for damaged and dry skin		100 percent
Carrot		Premature aging, dryness, itching, eczema, psoriasis, reduces scarring, rejuvenating,	Additive to a base, not exceeding 10 percent
Corn	All skin types		100 percent
Evening Primrose		Multiple sclerosis, menopausal problems, heart disease, eczema, psoriasis	Additive to a base, not exceeding 10 percent

Grapeseed	All skin types		100 percent
Hazelnut		has a slight astringent action	100 percent
Jojoba	All skin types	Inflamed skin, eczema, psoriasis, hair care, acne	Additive to a base, not exceeding 10 percent
Olive		Hair care, rheumatic conditions, soothing, cosmetics	Additive to a base, not exceeding 10 percent
Peanut	All skin types		100 percent
Safflower	All skin types		100 percent
Sesame	All skin types	Eczema, psoriasis, arthritis, rheumatism,	Additive to a base, not exceeding 10 percent
Soy Bean	All skin types		100 percent
Sunflower	All skin types		100 percent
Wheatgerm	All skin types, particularly premature aged skin	psoriasis, eczema,	Additive to a base, not exceeding 10 percent

As you have noticed from the list above, some carrier oils should never be used by themselves and are better blended with other carrier oils.

Massage Oils

Massage is a nourishing and relaxing experience in itself. It also allows the oils to be effectively absorbed through the skin and into the blood stream. Follow the ratio indicated below to mix your massage oil according to the amount you think you may need for your massage.

The Rule of the Thumb

For topical blends, a 2% dilution is the best way to mix essential and carrier oils.

- 10 drops essential oil or blend for every 30 ml carrier oil

Lotions and Skin Oils

You can prepare essential oil for lotions and skin oils in the same manner as massage oils. However, your base oil should include more nourishing oils, such as avocado, jojoba, and apricot kernel.

- If you have a bland lotion or cream, add a few drops of essential oil to boost it.
- Add a few drops to a basic facial mask, such as honey, oatmeal, or clay.
- For athlete's feet and cold sores, you can mix 6 drops of oil with 5 mil vodka or alcohol.
- For treating sores and open cuts, you can dilute the athlete's foot mix with a liter of boiled and cooled water.

How to Properly Apply

A gentle circular movement of the fingers is not sufficient for the oil to be absorbed. You need to drag on the skin, particularly in delicate areas, such as the neck and around the eyes.

Important Reminder

Never mix pure essential oils with carrier oil and then just store them away. The therapeutic property of the essential oil will rapidly break down with the vegetable protein of the carrier oil. Thus, leaving you with a low quality oil that does not smell as good.

Instead, mix according to the specified proper ratio indicated above only when needed.

Add To Bath

Distilled water is an excellent carrier for essential oils. Even plain bath water has astonishing results. Putting drops of oil into water imbues it with therapeutic properties. Moreover, it is believed that essential oil put in bath water enters the body via osmosis.

Bathtub

Add 2 to 5 drops of essential oil or blend to a tub filled with bath water. Enjoy a 10-minute soak.

Bath with Milk

Essential oil with milk is the perfect combination for your relaxing bath. Not only will it help you lose weight, it will also leave your skin smooth and nourished after.

Weight Loss Milk Bath

- 2 cups whole powdered milk
- 1/2 cup baking soda
- 1/2 cup cornstarch
- 10 drops of your preferred essential oil or blend

Directions:
1. Combine the milk, baking soda, and cornstarch in a large glass container.
2. Close the lid and shake the jar until the contents are mixed completely.
3. Open the lid. Add the drops of essential oil or blend. Re-cap and shake well to combine.
4. Allow to sit for 24 hours in a cool, dark place before using.
5. Pour about 1-2 cups of the mix into your tub under hot water. Soak and enjoy.

Foot Bath

This method will pull the toxins away from your body.
1. Add 2 to 5 drops of essential oil or blend into a large bowl filled with warm water.
2. Swish the mix around.

Jacuzzi or Hot Tub

Follow the same method used for bathtub.

Hot Shower

Pour a few drops in the bottom of the shower or the tub. The hot water will diffuse the essential oil in an upward manner. The upward draft will be absorbed by your feet and through the large pores. You can close the drain and allow 2-3 inches of water to build up if you are using a tub.

Aromatherapy Diffuser

Diffusion is subtle scenting of the air with the aroma of the essential oil. The result is a mild aromatherapy, breathing in the therapeutic properties of the oil indirectly into your system.

Oil Burner Diffusion

Remember that essential oils are highly flammable and could be dangerous. Make sure to place the burner in a safe area, away from any flammable material.

1.   Pour 5 drops of oil or blend into an oil dish.
2.   Fill the balance with warm water.
3.   Light the candle.
4.   Allow the flame to warm the bowl.
5.   Enjoy the dispersing aroma.

If you are going to leave the room for a long time, extinguish the flame.

Lamp Ring Diffusers

The heat from the light bulb will heat the oil or blend in the terra-cotta lamp ring, diffusing the aroma into the room.

Clay Pot Diffusers

This diffuser resembles small terra-cotta pots. It has an opening, usually opened and closed with a cork, where the oil or blend is added through. The aroma will permeate through and diffuse in the room.

Candle Diffuser

Usually glass, metal, or ceramic that uses a tea candle or light to gently heat the oil.

Fan Diffuser

This diffuser blows cool air through the essential oil pad, which releases the therapeutic benefits into the air.

Electric Heat Diffusers

This is similar to a fan diffuser. It heats the oil and fans the aroma to disperse into a room.

Chapter 5
Weight Loss Blends

Now comes the most important part of using essential oil to aid weight loss - blending to get that perfect aroma that you can enjoy while reaping the benefits. You can use an essential oil by itself or you can combine it with other oils to create blends. You can simply combine the same amount of Bergamot, Lemongrass, and Grapefruit essential oils together. In fact, I use this blend often. However, I also create different blends to enjoy.

Please note that you do not need to buy all the six best essential oils all at once. I had started with 2 bottles myself – lemon and grapefruit. Slowly, I added more bottles of essential oils until I had enough to mix various blends and aromas.

Start with a single, simple aroma and work your way up. A single bottle will last between 5-10 years.

Note Blending

Blending essential oils is not as simple as putting them all together. The key is to blend them in perfect harmony to create a pleasing fragrance that will suit your senses.

Top Notes	Middle (to Top) Notes	Middle Notes	Middle (to Base) Notes	Base
Anise	Angelica (seed)	Allspice	Angelica (root)	Amyris
Bergamot	Basil	Caraway	Benzoin	Birch
Cassia	Bay	Cardamom	Cananga	Frankincense
Fennel (sweet)	Cajeput	Carrot	Cedarwood	Labdanum
Hyssop	Camphor	Chamomile (r)	Chamomile (g)	Myrrh
Lavender (spike)	Catnip	**Cinnamon**	Clary sage	Oakmoss
Lemon	Celery	Clove	Cypress	Patchouli
Lime	Citronella	Coriander	Helichrysum	Sandalwood
Mandarin	Eucalyptus	Cumin	Jasmine	Spikenard
Orange (bitter)	*Grapefruit*	Dill	Lovage (root)	Storax
Peppermint	Lavandin	Elemi	Pepper	Turmeric
Petitgrain	Lemongrass	Fennel (bitter)	Rose (maroc)	Valerian
Rose (damask)	Litsea	Fir	Ylang-ylang	Vetiver
Sage (common)	Lovage (leaf/stalk)	Galangal		
Spearmint	Myrtle	Galbanum		
Spruce	Pine	Geranium		
Yarrow	Rosemary	Ginger		
	Tagetes	Hops		
	Tea tree	Juniper		
	Thyme	Lavender (true)		
		Orange (sweet)		
		Oregano		
		Palmarosa		
		Parsley		
		Sage (spanish)		
		Savory		
		Star anise		
		Lemon balm		
		Marjoram		
		Mugwort		
		Neroli		
		Niaouli		
		Nutmeg		

How to Blend Notes

Let's not get complicated with this. The simple rule of the thumb for blending essential for a wonderful fragrance is to blend in the following ratio:

- 3 drops top-middle notes
- 2 drops middle notes
- 1 drop base note

You can also reverse the formula if you want to emphasize the base note.

Choose an essential oil from the top and top to middle notes, add an essential oil from the middle and middle to base notes, and then complete your blend with essential oil from middle to base and base notes.

Remember, if you are going to use your blend for topical use, always dilute with a carrier or base oil.

Weight Loss Essential Oil Blends

Fat-Burning Massage Blend

Mix the following essential oils and add 10 drops of the blend into 30 ml carrier oil.

2 drops peppermint
1 drop lemon
3 drops German (blue) chamomile
2 drops ginger
4 drops lavender
2 drops cardamom

Directions:
Lightly cover the skin with the diluted blend. Massage in a light, gentle stroking circle motions.

Massage/Bath Oil

Mix the following essential oils and add 10 drops of the blend into 30 ml carrier oil.
5 drops peppermint EO
3 drops ginger EO
5 drops sweet marjoram EO
3 drops cypress EO

For a romantic effect, also add 8 drops of sandalwood EO

Aromatic Weight Loss Blend

2 ounces almond oil (carrier)
5 drops grapefruit EO
5 drops lemon EO
5 drops cypress EO

Anti-Cellulite Oil Rub

Blend the following recipe to your preferred carrier before using as massage oil.
10 drops grapefruit EO
5 drops rosemary EO
2 drops cypress EO
2 drops peppermint EO
2 drops ginger EO

Rejuvenating Bath Oil

Add the following to your warm bath.
5 drops grapefruit EO
5 drops ginger EO
5 drops orange EO
5 drops sandalwood EO
5 drops lemon EO

Appetite Suppressing Diffuser Blend

Mix together the following essential oils and then pour a few drops of the blend into your diffuser.
10 drops mandarin
5 drops lemon
3 drops ginger
3 drops peppermint

Appetite Curbing Salve

In a 30 ml carrier oil, add the following essential oils and then massage on your abdomen.
10 drops fennel EO
5 drops bergamot
3 drops patchouli

Simple Weight Loss Bath

Add 20 drops of any of the following fat-burning essential oils into your warm bath water.
Orange
Peppermint
Ginger
Basil
Rosemary
Lemon
Grapefruit

Weight Loss Bath Blend

In 1 cup of apple cider vinegar, add the following essential oils, and add to your warm bath.
5 drops grapefruit
5 drops ginger
5 drops orange
5 drops sandalwood
5 drops lemon

Directions:
Never add essential oil directly to running water to avoid evaporation. Mix the EO cider blend into the warm tub water by hand. Soak for 20-30 minutes.

Calming Weight Loss Bath Blend

3 drops geranium EO
3 drops lavender EO
2 drops lemon EO
2 drops sandalwood EO

Wake Up Weight Loss Bath Blend

5 drops rosemary EO
4 drops peppermint EO
3 drops bay EO
2 drops ginger EO

Winter Weight Loss Bath Blend

6 drops grapefruit EO
6 drops elemi EO
4 drops ginger EO
2 drops sandalwood EO

Moisturizing Anti-cellulite Body Oil

Basic Moisturizing Oil
Blend the following Oil and then add 20 drops of the anti-cellulite blend.
90 ml sweet almond oil
5 ml jojoba oil

Anti-Cellulite Blend

5 drops rosemary EO
5 drops lemon EO
4 drops fennel EO
2 drops ginger EO
2 drops cypress EO
2 drops juniper EO

Pain-Free Weight Loss Blend

If you want to create a blend to help you lose excess
weight and at the same time to cure body aches, just
mix the following essential oils.
10 drops lavender oil
8 drops rosemary
4 drops peppermint
4 drops ginger
4 drops black pepper

Muscle Toner Weight Loss Blend

8 drops grapefruit
4 drops ginger
3 drops lemon
3 drops cypress
2 drops juniper

Aromatic Weight Loss Room Spray

Mix 10ml vodka or alcohol and 10ml distilled water. (The vodka keeps the oils fresh and the water helps disperse it into the air.) Then, add 10 drops of your preferred blend from the choices below. Shake and then use to spray around the room.

Aromatic Weight Loss Body Spray

Mix 30 drops of your preferred bend into a 30 ml of distilled water. Spray the mix upward into the air and walk underneath. If the aroma is not strong enough, add 5-drop additions until to your desired strength. You can also use these blends for your bath drops, massage oil, or diffuser.

Festive Weight Loss Blend

6 drops orange
2 drops Ylang-Ylang
1 drop cinnamon
1 drop lemon

Romantic Holiday Weight Loss Blend

5 drops rose
3 drops Ylang-Ylang
2 drops patchouli
2 drops bergamot

Weight Loss Holiday Ambience Blend

15 drops fir needle
7 drops orange
7 drops black pepper
5 drops anise
5 drops cinnamon

Chapter 6
Essential Oil Safety and Precautions

When used correctly, essential oil is very safe to use for beauty and health purposes. However, even too much water can be detrimental to health. The key is to take the appropriate doses and prepare the various blends accordingly to their therapeutic uses. Although essential oils generally fall under natural remedies and supplements, they are chemically different and require their own set of safety guidelines and recommendations.

General Safety Rules

To ensure safe usage and to obtain the maximum health benefits of essential oil, follow these basic guides.

Store Them Safely

Keep bottles out of reach of pets and children. Essential oils are not like any other vitamin or herbal supplement.

Store Them Properly

Keep all your essential oil bottles tightly closed and store them in cool places, away from direct sunlight.

Never Apply Directly to Ears, Eyes, and Nose

Pure essential oils are highly concentrated and these parts of the body are highly sensitive to the reactions of essential oil, whether pure or diluted.

Always Buy High-Quality Oil

Buying pure, unadulterated, natural essential oils is vital for safety. Do not buy flavorings or fragrance. Most allergic reactions and adverse effects are due to the synthetic chemicals found in modified aromatic products.

Always Test for Sensitivity

Before using essential oil directly on your skin, test if you are sensitive to it.

Combine:

1 drop of essential oil

1/2 teaspoon of carrier oil (like jojoba, sweet almond, or olive)

Rub the dilution on the inside, upper portion of your arm. Wait for a few hours and inspect the area. If no itching of redness develops, then you are not sensitive to that particular essential oil.

Aromatic Use Safety Guidelines

Among the three primary uses of essential oil, (internal, topical, and aromatic) aromatic use is the safest. If you are going to diffuse essential oil around pets or young children, use smaller amounts, especially if you are using known irritating oils, such as cinnamon bark.

Internal Use Safety Guidelines

Taking essential oil orally or internally is the most risky use. When taken in high doses, compounds of certain essential oils can cause liver damage. Avoid using oils that are high in phenols and ethers. Using only for a short time or a few days will minimize the risk of overworking the liver.

It is not recommended to ingest pure essential oils daily and taking oil orally should only be under the supervision of a trained aromatherapist or a medical professional.

Topical Use Safety Guidelines

The golden safety rule for essential oil topical use is to DILUTE. Using pure essential oil can cause irritation, phototoxic reactions, and sensitization, as well as systemic toxicities.

Avoid Sensitization and Irritation

Irritation is a localized, temporary effect that can be caused by pure essential oil and is often recognized by itching and redness. On the other hand, sensitization is an immune reaction of the body exposed to the oil, which can show up only during the second or later application or exposure to the oil. Both irritation and sensitization can be avoided by proper dilution.

Prevent Oxidation

Proper storage of essential oil is important. Oxidation from light can make the oil not just less effective, but also irritating. Always make sure to tightly close the lid after using and to store the bottles away from light and in a cool place.

Avoid Phototoxicity

Some essential oils contain compounds that cause them to react to light (particularly UV light), which can cause burns and discolorations on the skin. These oils can generally be used aromatically, in wash off products, or in skin areas that are covered with clothes. Dilution also makes these essential oil safe for topical applications.

Phototoxicity Safety Guide

Listed below are the most commonly used phototoxic oil. Follow the recommended drop of each for every 30 ml or 1 ounce of carrier oil for safe use.

1 drop Bergamot (Citrus bergamia)

12 drops lemon (Citrus limon)

4 drops lime (Citrus aurantifolia)

24 drops grapefruit (Citrus paradisi)

Dilute, Dilute, Dilute!

Diluting is the most effective method to avoid long-term and short-term negative dermal reactions while retaining the essential oil's therapeutic benefits.

Thank You

Thank you so much for reading this book. I hope it has helped and encouraged you.

If you enjoyed it, I would really appreciate if you could take a minute of your time and leave me a review on Amazon.

It helps a bunch and I personally read every single review. Thanks again and best of luck to you on your weight loss journey.

www.ingramcontent.com/pod-product-compliance
Lightning Source LLC
Chambersburg PA
CBHW062117280526
45788CB00003B/1500